# REASONS TO CIRCUMCISE:

## A COMPREHENSIVE UNBIASED EVIDENCE-BASED GUIDE TO ALL OF THE DATA IN FAVOR OF CIRCUMCISION

By

Hugh Dickman, M.D.



KPD ISBN: 9781651834305

*"Primum non nocerum."*
*(First, do no harm.)*

— Hippocrates

# CONTENTS

CHAPTER 1

# MEDICINE

# Reasons To Circumcise

# Reasons To Circumcise

CHAPTER 2
# RELIGION

25

35

43

# CHAPTER 3
# HEALTH

49

52

56

CHAPTER 4
# PARENTING

CHAPTER 5

# SEXUALITY

75

85

87

CHAPTER 6
# CHOICE

CHAPTER 7
# APPEARANCE

CHAPTER 8
# CULTURE

CHAPTER 9
# VALUES

142

# FURTHER RESOURCES

American Circumcision (Documentary Film) CircumcisionMovie.com

## ABOUT THE AUTHOR

155

Hugh Dickman, M.D. is an obvious pseudonym.

9 781651 834305